God gifted inside everyone self-healing mechanism. My vision is not only to increase awareness about Varicocele but to activate the vital force to access self natural healing of the body.

A	What is a varicocele?
B	What causes a varicocele to develop?
C	Recognizing the symptoms of a varicocele
D	Possible complications
E	How is a varicocele diagnosed?
F	Methods of treatment for varicoceles.
G	Varicocele embolization
H	Living with a varicocele.
I	Most effective Homeopathic medicine for varicoceles.
J	Ayurvedic Approach in Varicocele
K	Summary about Varicocele

INDEX

<u>Varicocele</u>

A. What is a varicocele?

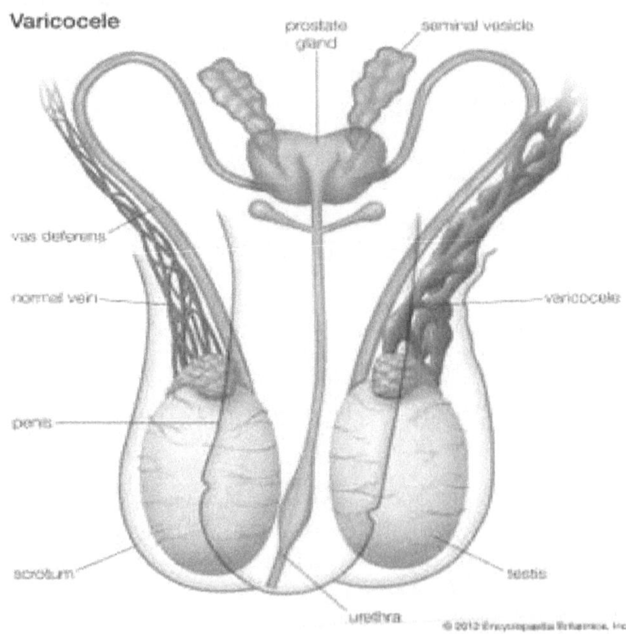

Varicocele, pronounced "vari-co-seel," is when veins in your scrotum swell and get enlarged. It's a lot like a varicose vein in your leg. It might feel like a bag of worms.

It usually shows up above one your testicles, most often the left one. You can usually see it when you stand up, but not when you lie down.

It should be harmless, but it can be uncomfortable or painful. And it might affect your fertility or cause your testicles to shrink.

This condition is fairly common and usually affects young men. About 10 to 15 of every 100 men have this problem.

If your varicocele causes problems, your doctor may send you to a specialist called a urologist.

The scrotum is a skin-covered sac that holds your testicles. It also contains the arteries and veins that deliver blood to the reproductive glands. A vein abnormality in the scrotum may result in a varicocele. A varicocele is an enlargement of the veins within the scrotum. These veins are called the pampiniform plexus.

A varicocele only occurs in the scrotum and is very similar to varicose veins that can occur in the leg.

A varicocele can result in decreased sperm production and quality, which in some cases can lead to infertility. It can also shrink the testicles.

Varicoceles are graded into:

- **Grade III**: When the distended venous plexus bulges visibly through the scrotal skin and is easily palpable.

- **Grade II**: When the intrascrotal venous distension is easily palpable but not visible.

- **Grade I**: When there is no visible or palpable distension except when the man performs the Valsalva manoeuvre.

- **Subclinical**: Where there is no clinical varicocele but an abnormality is present upon scrotal thermography or duplex Doppler ultrasonography

Table. Baseline Characteristics

Parameter	Overall	Hypogonadism	Pain	p value
Number, (%)	29	14 (48.3)	15 (51.7)	
Age, median (IQR)	33 (19)	41.5 (18)	29 (22)	0.051[a]
Baseline Testosterone (ng/dL), mean (SD)	308.6 (75.9)	270.6 (62.8)	344.1 (71.2)	0.007[b]
Bilateral Varicocele, n (%)	14 (48.3)	8 (57.1)	6 (40.0)	0.466[c]
Left Varicocele Grade				0.365[c]
1, n (%)	2 (6.9)	0 (0)	2 (13.3)	
2, n (%)	6 (20.7)	3 (21.4)	3 (20.0)	
3, n (%)	21 (72.4)	11 (78.6)	10 (66.7)	
Right Varicocele Grade				0.534[c]
0, n (%)	15 (51.7)	6 (42.9)	9 (60.0)	
1, n (%)	4 (13.8)	2 (14.3)	2 (13.3)	
2, n (%)	7 (24.1)	5 (35.7)	2 (13.3)	
3, n (%)	3 (10.3)	1 (7.1)	2 (13.3)	
Left Testis Volume (cc), median (IQR)	18 (5)	19 (10)	15 (5)	0.867[a]
Right Testis Volume (cc), median (IQR)	20 (7)	21 (8)	18 (4)	0.583[a]

Abbreviations: IQR - Interquartile range, SD - Standard deviation

Tests: [a]Rank sum test, [b]Student's t test, [c]Chi squared test

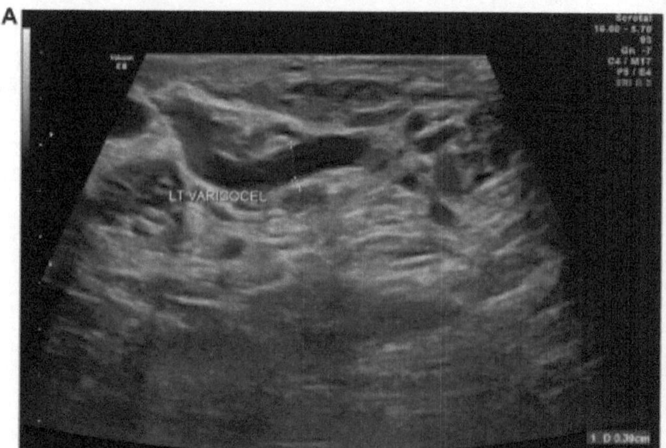
A
LT VARICOCEL

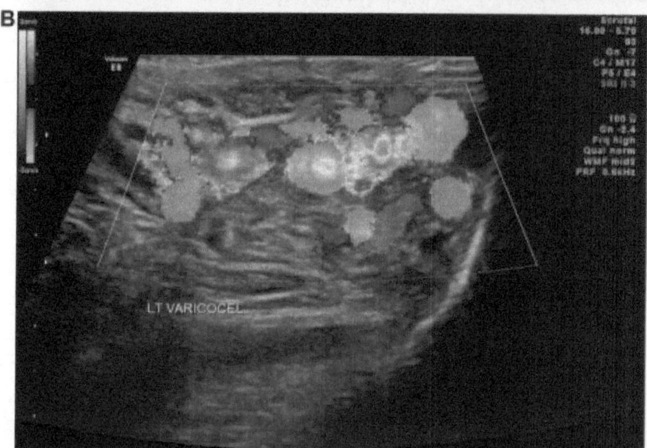
B
LT VARICOCEL

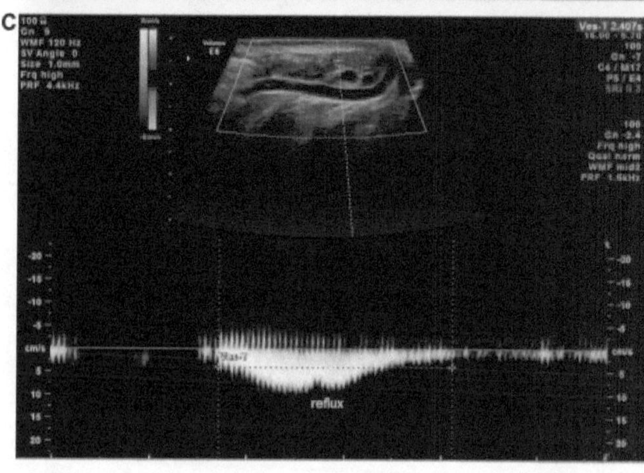
C
reflux

Varicoceles are common. They can be found in 15 percent of the adult male population and around 20 percent of adolescent males. They're more common in males aged 15 to 25.

Varicoceles generally form during puberty and are more commonly found on the left side of your scrotum. The anatomy of the right and left side of your scrotum isn't the same. Varicoceles can exist on both sides, but it's extremely rare. Not all varicoceles affect sperm production.

Variable	Total testosterone level		P-value
	≥ 3 ng/ml	< 3 ng/ml	
Age			< 0.005
30–39	138 (80.2)	34 (19.8)	
40–49	151 (65.7)	79 (34.3)	
50–59	182 (63.0)	107 (37.0)	
60–70	192 (54.7)	159 (45.3)	
Income			< 0.005
< 500	290 (55.8)	230 (44.2)	
≥ 500	373 (71.5)	149 (28.5)	
Education			< 0.005
Less than university	255 (56.3)	198 (43.7)	
University	408 (69.3)	181 (30.7)	
Body mass index (kg/m^2)			< 0.004
< 25	120 (70.6)	50 (29.4)	
Overweight	276 (66.7)	138 (33.3)	
Obese	267 (58.3)	191 (41.7)	
Smoking			
Non-smoker	179 (64.9)	97 (35.1)	0.004
Past-smoker	178 (58.0)	129 (42.0)	
Current	306 (66.7)	379 (36.4)	
Hypertension			0.055
Yes	536 (62.5)	322 (37.5)	
No	127 (69.0)	57 (31.0)	
Dyslipidemia			0.493
Yes	612 (63.7)	349 (36.3)	
No	51 (63.0)	30 (37.0)	
Diabetic retinopathy (DR)			0.002
No DR	249 (69.9)	107 (30.1)	
Non proliferative DR	364 (61.7)	226 (38.3)	
Proliferative DR	50 (52.1)	46 (47.9)	
Diabetic nephropathy			0.070
Yes	217 (60.4)	142 (39.6)	
No	446 (65.3)	237 (34.7)	
Diabetic neuropathy			< 0.005
Yes	210 (54.4)	176 (45.6)	
No	453 (69.1)	203 (30.9)	
Duration of diabetes			< 0.005
≤ 5 years	339 (70.3)	143 (29.7)	
6–10 years	168 (65.1)	90 (34.9)	
> 10 years	156 (51.7)	146 (48.3)	
HbA1c			
HbA1C ≤ 7	158 (70.5)	66 (29.5)	0.009
HbA1C > 7	505 (61.7)	313 (38.3)	

B. What causes a varicocele to develop?

A spermatic cord holds up each testicle. The cords also contain the veins, arteries, and nerves that support these glands. In healthy veins inside the scrotum, one-way valves move the blood from the testicles to the scrotum, and then they send it back to the heart.

Sometimes the blood doesn't move through the veins like it should and begins to pool in the vein, causing it to enlarge. A varicocele develops slowly over time.

There are no established risk factors for developing a varicocele, and the exact cause is unclear.

C. Recognizing the symptoms of a varicocele

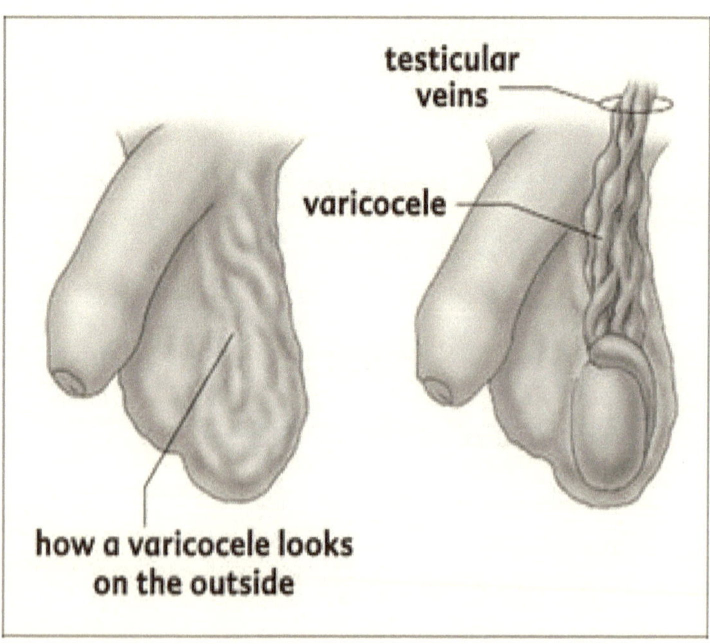

Varicoceles rarely hurt. You may not even know you have one until you or the doctor sees it.

If yours does cause pain, it might:

- ✓ Switch from dull to sharp
- ✓ Get worse when you stand or exert yourself, especially for a long time
- ✓ Become more intense as the day goes on
- ✓ Go away when you lie on your back

Group	Recurrence/No. of varicoceles			p-value*
	Grade I	Grade II	Grade III	
1	1/16 (6.3)	3/29 (10.3)	4/28 (14.3)	<0.05
2	0/12 (0)	2/14 (14.3)	3/12 (25)	<0.05
3	0/14 (0)	1/16 (6.3)	3/15 (20)	<0.05

knowledge question	Number (%)
Varicocele definition	
Dilatation of testicular veins	172 (76.4)
Others	
Testicular inflammation	29 (12.9)
Absent testis	7 (3.1)
Testicular torsion	13 (5.8)
Others	4 (1.8)
Varicocele most common symptom	
Dull recurrent testicular pain	177 (78.7)
Back pain	19 (8.4)
Scrotal rash	9 (4)
Scrotal itching	15 (6.7)
Others	5 (2.2)
Relation of varicocele to infertility	
Yes	157 (69.8)
No	68 (30.2)

You may have no symptoms associated with a varicocele. However, you might experience:

- ✓ A lump in one of your testicles
- ✓ Swelling in your scrotum
- ✓ Visibly enlarged or twisted veins in your scrotum, which are often described as looking like a bag of worms
- ✓ A dull, recurring pain in your scrotum

D. Possible complications

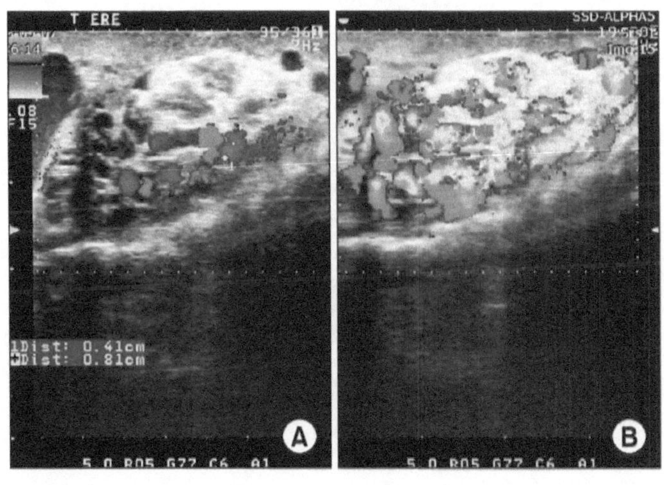

This condition can have an effect on fertility. Varicocele is present in 35 to 44 percent of men with primary infertility and in 45 to 81 percent of men with secondary infertility.

Primary infertility is generally used to refer to a couple that hasn't conceived a child after at least one year of trying. Secondary infertility describes couples that have conceived at least once but aren't able to again.

E. How is a varicocele diagnosed?

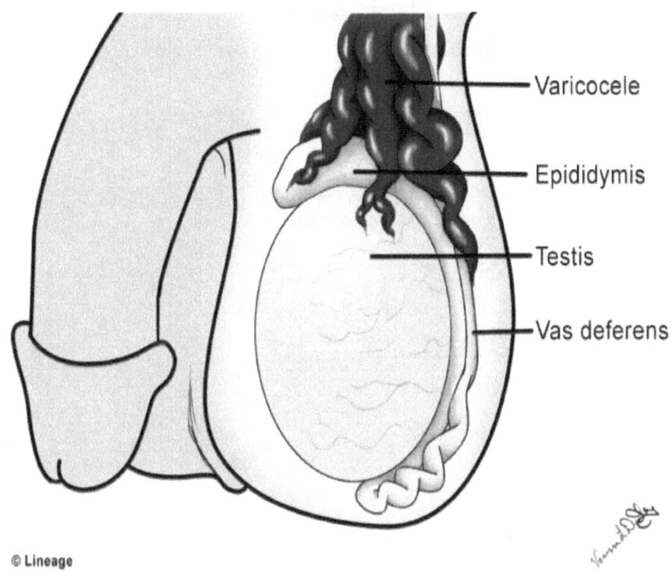

Your doctor usually diagnoses the condition after a physical exam. A varicocele can't always be felt or seen when you're lying down. Your doctor will most likely examine your testicles while you're standing up and lying down.

Your doctor may need to perform a scrotal ultrasound. This helps measure the spermatic veins and allows your doctor to get a detailed, accurate picture of the condition.

Once the varicocele is diagnosed, your doctor will classify it with one of three clinical grades. They're labeled grades 1 through 3, according to the size of the lump in your testicle. Grade 1 is the smallest and grade 3 the largest.

The size doesn't necessarily affect the overall treatment because you may not require treatment. Treatment options are based on the degree of discomfort or infertility issues you have.

F. Methods of treatment for varicoceles.

It's not always necessary to treat a varicocele. However, you may want to consider treatment if the varicocele:

- ➢ causes pain
- ➢ causes testicular atrophy
- ➢ causes infertility

You may also want to consider treatment if you're thinking about assisted reproductive techniques.

This condition can cause problems with testicular functioning in some people. The earlier you start treatment, the better your chances of improving sperm production.

Wearing tight underwear or a jock strap can sometimes provide you with support that alleviates pain or discomfort. Additional treatment, such as varicocelectomy and varicocele embolization, might be necessary if your symptoms get worse.

G. Varicocele embolization

Varicocele embolization is a less invasive, same-day procedure. A small catheter is inserted into a groin or neck vein. A coil is then placed into the catheter and into the varicocele. This blocks blood from getting to the abnormal veins.

H. Living with a varicocele.

Infertility is a common complication of a varicocele. Talk to your doctor about seeing a reproductive specialist if you and your partner are having problems getting pregnant.

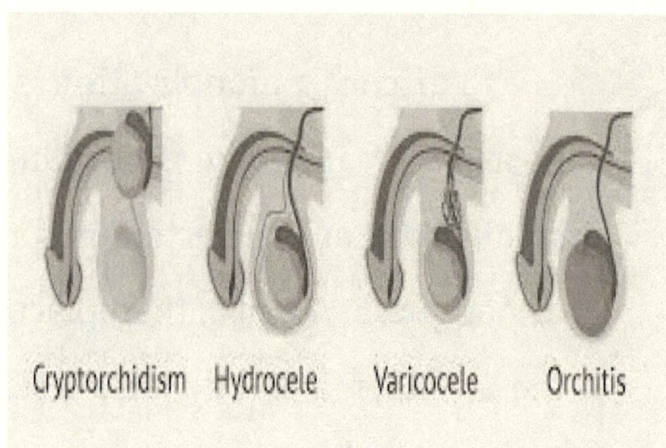

Cryptorchidism
Hydrocele
Varicocele
Orchitis

I. Most effective Homeopathic Substance for varicocele.

Sr. No	Healing Substance	Power	Formula	Doses
1	Hamamelis	30	Mix 10 ml of each in a new Bottle	15 Drops with ½ cup of water 3 times a day
2	Aesculus	30		
3	Belladonna	30		
4	Calcium Fluoratum	30		
5	Carduus Marianus	200		
6	Mezereum	200		
7	Placenta (Suis)	30		
8	Pulsatilla	30		
9	Secale comutum	30		
10	Vipera Berus	200		
11	CALCAREA FLUORICA	6 X	4 (Tablets) 3 Times a day	
12	Thuja	200	4 Drops morning daily	
13	Hamamelis	30	3 Drops morning and evening daily empty stomach	
14	Hamamelis	Q	15 Drops with ½ cup of water,	

			3 times a day

Ayurvedic Approach in Varicocele

Note (1):- Salad of one onion, two tomato, one **green chilli (Necessary)** mixing with half lemon have great healing property in case of Varicocele & other symptoms also. **(Take it also with Homeopathic treatment)**

Note (2):- Flex seeds & Cinnamon in very few quantity is also helpful ingredients for varicocele.

Note (3):- 2 Green Chilli with Salad or food makes blood flow easy in dilated veins.

Thanking You